Fatma Chaker
Mohamed Derbel
Fatma Khanfir

The effect of dystocic childbirth on women's psychology

Fatma Chaker
Mohamed Derbel
Fatma Khanfir

The effect of dystocic childbirth on women's psychology

ScienciaScripts

Imprint

Cover image: www.ingimage.com

This book is a translation from the original published under ISBN 978-620-6-71125-4.

Publisher:
Sciencia Scripts
is a trademark of
Dodo Books Indian Ocean Ltd. and OmniScriptum S.R.L publishing group

120 High Road, East Finchley, London, N2 9ED, United Kingdom
Str. Armeneasca 28/1, office 1, Chisinau MD-2012, Republic of Moldova, Europe
Printed at: see last page
ISBN: 978-620-7-61664-0

TABLE OF CONTENTS

INTRODUCTION

Pregnancy and childbirth are significant events in a woman's life. The experience is often idealised and seen by society as a source of happiness. However, for women, childbirth can be an extremely stressful event, both expected and feared. Aktaet al. have reported childbirth as a multidimensional experience in which pain, stress, sadness, happiness and joy are associated(1) .

Under physiological conditions, childbirth is uncomplicated for both mother and baby. However, certain circumstances can lead to a difficult or dystocic birth. These may include prolonged labour, an emergency caesarean section (to save the mother and/or foetus), an instrumental extraction to speed up or facilitate delivery, and/or an immediate post-partum complication such as haemorrhage.

Childbirth, particularly dystocic childbirth, can be a traumatic experience for women(2,3) . In the postnatal period, women may be vulnerable to a wide variety of psychiatric disorders. Indeed, a negative experience of childbirth has been reported to be predictive of post-partum depression or post-traumatic stress disorder(4,5) . These conditions can have as much impact on the mother-baby relationship as on the marital relationship(6,7) .

As a result, particular attention needs to be paid to the psychological environment of post-partum women, especially following a dystocic birth. Screening for situations where there is a risk of psychological impact would enable childbirth-related psychiatric disorders to be managed appropriately and avoid their psychological, economic and social repercussions.
The primary objectives of our study were:

- To assess the intensity of post-traumatic stress disorder and depression in the post-partum in patients with dystocic delivery.

- To determine the factors associated with post-traumatic stress disorder and post-partum depression in cases of dystocic childbirth.

- To assess the quality of the mother-baby relationship and the marital relationship in these patients.

The secondary objectives of our study were:

- To assess the epidemiological and obstetric characteristics and the experience of childbirth in patients with dystocic labour.

- Propose solutions to minimise the psychosocial impact of dystocic delivery in these patients.

THEORETICAL FRAMEWORK

I. Normal delivery and eutocic delivery :

According to the World Health Organisation (WHO)[8] , childbirth

physiological childbirth:

- spontaneously triggered.
- Low-risk from the start and throughout labour and delivery.
- Whose child (simple delivery) is born spontaneously in the vertex cephalic position, between 37ème and 42ème weeks of gestation or pregnancy;
- The post-partum evolution of the mother and child is normal. However, the i is necessary to However, it is necessary to differentiate between"normal physiological childbirth" and "eutoctal childbirth". In fact, a high-risk delivery may turn out to be eutoctal (normal delivery despite a pre-existing risk)[9] . In addition, medical interventions (analgesia, uterotonics, etc.) that interfere with physiological childbirth may be considered during an eutoctal birth.

II. Childbirth dystocic

Dystocia is defined as any phenomenon that interferes with the normal physiological process of childbirth. These phenomena may concern the mother (pelvis, uterine dynamics) and/or the foetus (position, presentation, volume).

1. Maternal dystocia :

They are explained by abnormalities in the parturient's body and are of two types:

- Mechanical dystocia: affects the bony structure of the pelvis, such as abnormalities in size, shape or inclination. Some dystocies are linked to the maternal genital tract and affect the soft tissues (10,11).

• Dynamic dystocies: these are all phenomena linked to dysfunction of the uterine "motor" or dilation of the cervix during labour, either due to a defect in uterine contractions which do not appear normal, or due to the ineffectiveness of apparently correct uterine contractions on dilation. There are 3 main groups of dynamic dystocies: a group linked to the uterine cervix (pathological cervix), a group linked to a primary or secondary pathology of uterine contraction (hypokinesia, hyperkinesia, hypertonia) and a group resulting in abnormalities in the dilatation curve (start-up dystocies, slow dilatation or cessation of dilatation). [(12).]

2. Fetal dystocia :

Fetal dystocia is the anomaly most frequently found in maternity wards. It can be explained by foetal macrosomia or by a presentation anomaly (breech, front, face, transverse presentation). Fetal dystocia can occur as a result of fetal-pelvic disproportion, shoulder dystocia or an abnormal position of the baby (breech or transverse presentation)[(13)] .

III. Instrumental delivery :

Instrumental extraction is defined as the use of an appropriate instrument (forceps, spatulas or suction cup) to give birth to a live child by the natural route in response to an unexpected situation of varying urgency, and requires the active participation of the patient (unless there are contraindications to expulsive efforts) after being informed. Its aim is to shorten the expulsion phase and to help flexion and/or complete rotation of the foetal head. The indications for an instrumental extraction may be fetal (poor tolerance of the fetus during labour), maternal (pre-existing factors - or not - in the pregnancy, insufficient expulsive efforts) or related to the delivery (obstructed labour). of the baby's progress due to the anatomy of the pelvic tract, for example)[(14,15)] .

Instrumental extractions are not harmless; they can increase the risk of anal sphincter tears (0.1% to 10.2%), vaginal tears, post-partum haemorrhage, acute urinary retention or anal incontinence in the year following an extraction in the mother. In the long term, these complications can lead to dyspareunia, sexual problems and perineal pain, sometimes even anal incontinence. In addition to the complications mentioned above, women may suffer psychological sequelae of childbirth, as instrumental extraction can be traumatic, and the lack of information may explain the anxiety-inducing nature of the procedure[16] .

In babies, instrumental extraction can be responsible for a number of neonatal complications, particularly in the head and neck area, such as intra- and extra-cranial haemorrhage, cephalohaematomas and facial nerve damage, especially when a suction cup is used, skull fractures with the risk of embarrure (in the case of forceps), retinal haemorrhage, poor adaptation to life outside the womb and often feeding difficulties. (17).

IV. Caesarean section :

A caesarean section is the surgical removal of a child by abdominal incision of the lower part of the uterus, when natural childbirth is not possible. It can be performed under general anaesthetic or spinal anaesthetic. A caesarean section can be scheduled, performed as an emergency or during labour. after an attempted natural birth (vaginal delivery).

• Scheduled caesarean section: this may be offered if there are foreseeable difficulties in the delivery that are likely to have consequences for the baby or the mother, or when vaginal delivery is contraindicated. A caesarean section may be scheduled in certain cases: an overlying placenta previa, a bi-healed uterus or more, transverse presentation of the foetus, severe diabetes with macrosomia, malignant disease of the mother, any foetal malformations that contraindicate vaginal delivery, foetopelvic disproportion and all gynaecological pathologies that make vaginal delivery impossible.

• Emergency caesarean section: this is indicated in emergency cases to save the mother or the baby, such as severe pre-eclampsia, Hellp Syndrome, retroplacental haematoma, uterine rupture (or suspected uterine rupture), or a threat of severe premature delivery that cannot allow vaginal delivery to proceed (after multidisciplinary discussion).

- Caesarean section during labour: a number of dystocia may require a caesarean section during labour (stagnation of dilatation or failure to achieve full dilatation, pathological foetal heart rate, failure of instrumental extraction, procidence of the cord in the case of cephalic presentation or in the case of podalic presentation with full dilatation, abnormality of presentation, etc.)(18,19,20)

.

V. The post-partum period :

The postnatal period is defined as the period from childbirth to six weeks afterwards (42 days). This is a critical period for patients, newborns, partners and relatives. Many psychological imbalances may arise. The mother may also experience strong and contradictory emotions such as joy, excitement, sadness, confusion and fatigue, which can have an impact on the mother's mental health and may be the cause of psychological problems.

1. Short-term mental disorders :

1.1.The baby blues :

It is a common and normal emotional reaction that can occur at any time after childbirth, but usually occurs in the first few days or weeks after giving birth. It affects approximately 50 to 80% of women give birth(21) . It is associated with mood swings, emotional sensitivity, fatigue, anxiety and frequent tears. It generally lasts for 4 to 5 days(22) . The baby blues can be caused by hormonal disturbances, parenthood problems, changes in lifestyle and the stress of post-natal recovery.

1.2.Puerperal psychosis :

A rare but serious mental disorder that can develop in some women after the birth of their child. It generally appears between five and twenty-five days after childbirth[23] . It is also known as post-partum psychosis and is characterised by symptoms such as hallucinations, delusions, confusion, agitation, unstable mood, insomnia and disorientation.

Women suffering from psychosis may experience delusions or suicidal ideation, leaving them unable to care for themselves or their children. It occurs 1 to 2 times per 1,000 pregnant women[24] .

2. Long-term mental disorders :

2.1. Post-partum depression :

It is a mood disorder characterised by depressive symptoms such as sadness, anxiety, weariness, sleep disturbance, anorexia, low mood and difficulty concentrating. According to the fifth edition of the Diagnostic and Statistical Manual of Mental Disorders (DSM-IV), PPD is a major depression that appears within 5 weeks of childbirth[25] , but can last up to a year. It affects between 15% and 20% of women who give birth. It can be caused by hormonal changes, sleep problems, predisposition to depression or anxiety, stress factors related to pregnancy and childbirth, and problems with social or family support.

Post-partum depression is under-diagnosed and under-treated, despite its serious consequences for the mother and, above all, for the child's mental, emotional and social development.

2.2. Post-traumatic stress disorder :

Post-traumatic stress disorder (PTSD) is a specific reaction that can develop in a person who has witnessed or been exposed to one or more traumatic events such as a sexual assault, a car accident, an act of terrorism or military combat. According to the DSM-5 diagnostic criteria, post-traumatic stress includes: reliving, avoidance, negative cognitions and mood, and hyper-reactivity[26] .

PTSD can be diagnosed as early as one month after exposure to the traumatic event.

PTSD can be associated with co-existing mental disorders, such as depression and anxiety disorders.

MATERIALS AND METHODS

I. Equipment

1. Type of study :

This was a descriptive and analytical cross-sectional study, conducted from 19 February 2023 to 19 March 2023 and including women who had given birth in the maternity ward of the Hedi Chaker University Hospital Centre (CHU) in Sfax during a period from 01 July 2022 to 31 December 2022.

2. Study population :

In order to obtain a homogeneous population, we established inclusion and non-inclusion criteria.

2.1.Inclusion criteria :

We included in our study women who had had a dystocic delivery for at least 3 months. We defined dystocic delivery as :

- Emergency caesarean section for abnormal labour.
- Instrumental delivery.
- A vaginal delivery complicated by shoulder dystocia

2.1.Non-inclusion criteria :

We did not include :

- Uncomplicated eutocic vaginal deliveries.
- Scheduled caesarean sections and emergency caesarean sections performed outside labour.
- Deliveries with a dystocic presentation, such as breech, forehead and transverse presentations.
- Births less than 3 months old.

- Women with a history of psychiatric pathology, a history of depression or post-traumatic stress disorder before giving birth.

- premature deliveries -single mothers.

-women who could not be contacted or who refused to take part in the survey.

3. Sample size :

During our study period, we enrolled 60 women who met the inclusion criteria in the maternity department of the Hédi Chaker University Hospital in Sfax.

II. Methods :

1. Data collection :

Initially, the patients' personal and medical data were collected from birth registers and obstetric records in the gynaecology-obstetrics department of the Hedi Chaker University Hospital in Sfax.

Secondly, we conducted a telephone interview with the women after obtaining their consent to take part in the study.

We drew up a data collection form comprising :

1.1. Data collected from medical records :

We reported information on the patient (age, history, gestational age and parity), the course of the pregnancy in question, the duration of labour, any emergency caesarean section or instrumental extraction, their indications and any post-partum complications.

1.2. The questionnaire:

It was an anonymous questionnaire written in French and translated into Arabic during the telephone interview. The questionnaire made it possible to report :

- identification of the woman (7 items)

- experience of current pregnancy (6 items)

- The woman's experience of childbirth (8items)

- Experiences of the post-partum period (2items)

- Changes in the mother-baby relationship, the marital relationship and family relationships after childbirth (7 items)

1.3.Edinburgh Postnatal Depression Scale (Appendix 1) To assess postnatal depression, we used the validated Arabic version of the Edinburgh Postnatal Depression Scale[27,28] .

This scale has 10 items. For each item, the closest response to what the participant felt is underlined.

The response categories are marked 0, 1, 2 and 3.

Items 1, 2 and 4 are marked 0, 1, 2 and 3.

Items 3, 5, 6, 7, 8, 9 and 10 are marked 3, 2, 1 and 0.

The total is calculated by adding up the results for the ten items. A cut-off of 13 or more was allowed for the validated Arabic version[28] .

1.4.The post-traumatic stress disorder scale (Appendix 2) :

To assess post-traumatic stress after childbirth, we used the IMPACT OF EVENTS SCALE- Revised (IES-R)[29] , translated into Arabic.

This scale comprises 22 items. It is divided into 3 sub-scales of post-traumatic symptoms:

Reviviscence (8 items): 1, 2, 3, 6, 9, 14, 16, 20

Avoidance (8 items): 5, 7, 8, 11, 12, 13, 17, 22

Psychophysiological activation (6 items): 4, 10, 15, 18, 19, 21[30] .

Each item is scored from 0 ("not at all") to 4 ("extremely"). The total is calculated by adding up the results for all the items. Scores range from 0 to 88, with a cut-off of 33 or more.

2. Ethical considerations :

We obtained the free consent of the participants by informing them of the aims of our study before beginning data collection.

3. Data entry and analysis :

The completed forms were entered into SPSS (Statistical Package for the Social Sciences) version 20. For quantitative variables, the means were estimated with their standard deviations and the medians with their minimum and maximum values, after verifying the normality of the distribution using the Kolmogorov-Smirnov test. Qualitative variables were expressed as numbers and percentages. For the analytical study, univariate and multivariate logistic regression models were used to study correlations. The threshold for statistical significance was set at a p-value of less than 0.05.

RESULTS

I. Descriptive study

1. Characteristics of parturients

1.1. Age

The mean age of our parturients was 29.1 years, with a standard deviation of 4.6 [19-40 years]. The distribution of parturients by age group is shown in Figure 1.

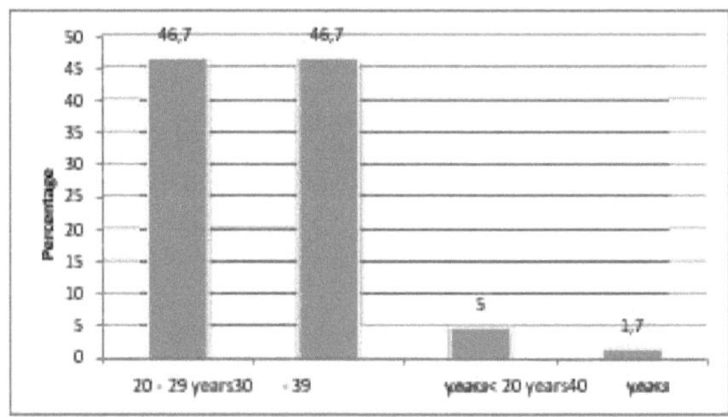

Figure 1: Distribution of parturients by age group.

1.2. Origin

Our parturients were of urban origin in 42 cases (70%) and of rural origin in 18. cases (30%) (Figure 2).

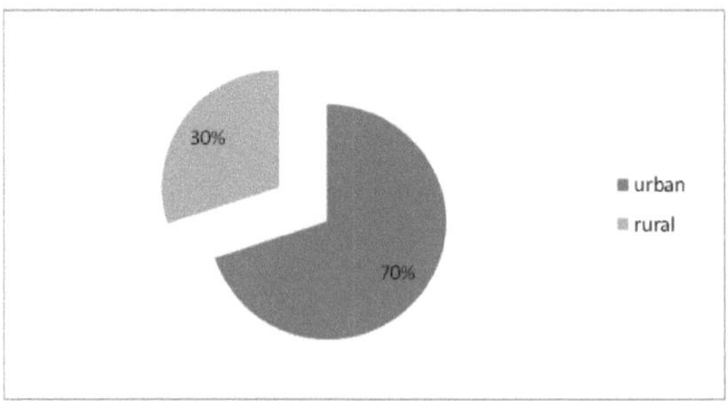

Figure 2: Distribution of parturients by origin

1.3.Level of study

The parturients had completed their secondary education in 45% of cases (Figure 3).

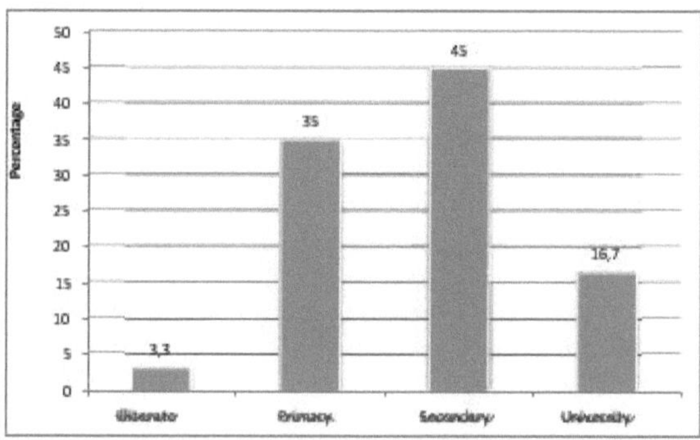

Figure 3: Distribution of parturients by level of education.

1.4. Situation

Housewives represented 56.7% of the series (Figure 4).

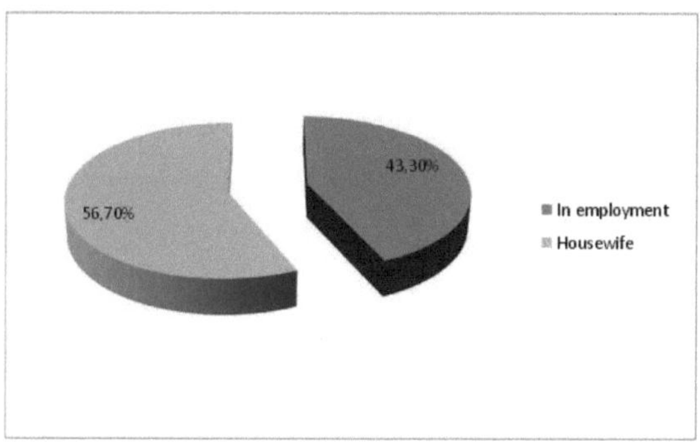

Figure 4: Distribution of parturients by professional status.

1.5.Socio-economic level

The majority of parturients (90%) were of average socio-economic status (Figure 5).

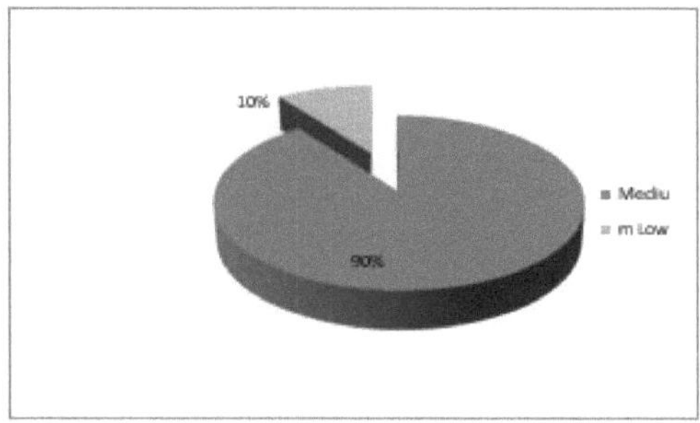

Figure 5: Distribution of parturients according to socio-economic level.

2. Gynaecological and obstetric history of parturients

2.1.Gestité and parity :

The primigravida represented 65% of the series. In addition primiparous in 71.7% of cases (Figure 6).

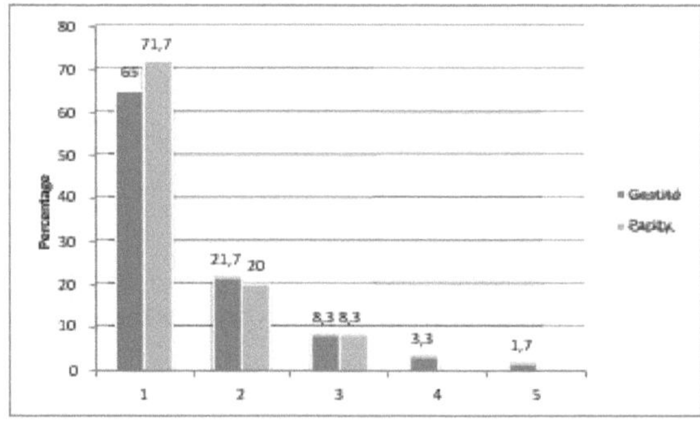

Figure 6: Distribution of parturients according to gestational age and parity.

2.2. Gynaecological history :

The gynaecological history of our parturients is shown in Table I.

Table I: Distribution of parturients according to gynaecological history.

	Workforce	Percentage
Spontaneous miscarriage	7	11,7%
Extra uterine pregnancy	1	1,7%
Fetal death in utero	1	1,7%

2.3.Judgement of previous births :

Of 17 parturients who had had a previous birth, 10 felt satisfied with their birth experience, 4 felt their birth was unsatisfactory and 3 were dissatisfied.

3. Characteristics of the current pregnancy :

3.1 Pregnancy :

Pregnancy was desired in the majority of cases (81.7%) (Figure 7).

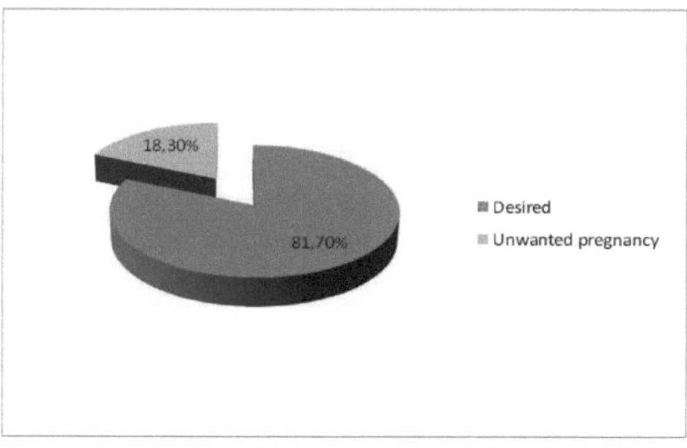

Figure 7: Distribution of parturients according to desire for pregnancy.

3.2.Pregnancy follow-up :

The pregnancy was well monitored in 76.7% of cases (Figure 8).

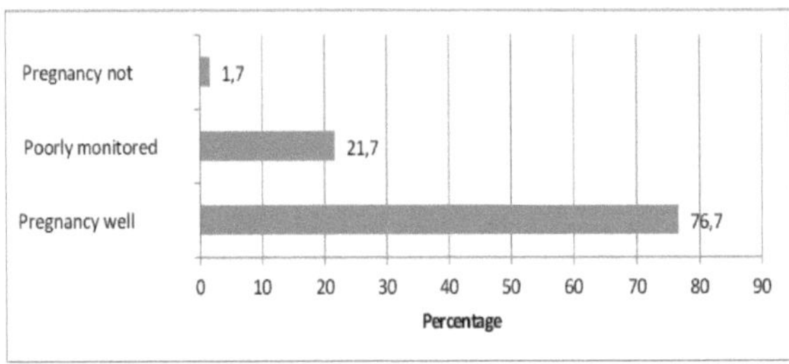

Figure 8: Distribution of parturients according to pregnancy follow-up.

3.3.Birth preparation :

Not all the parturients interviewed had attended birth preparation sessions.

3.4.Sources of information on childbirth :

The sources of information about the birth reported were the women's family and friends in almost half of cases (48.3%). No information was obtained for 18.3% of parturients (Figure 9).

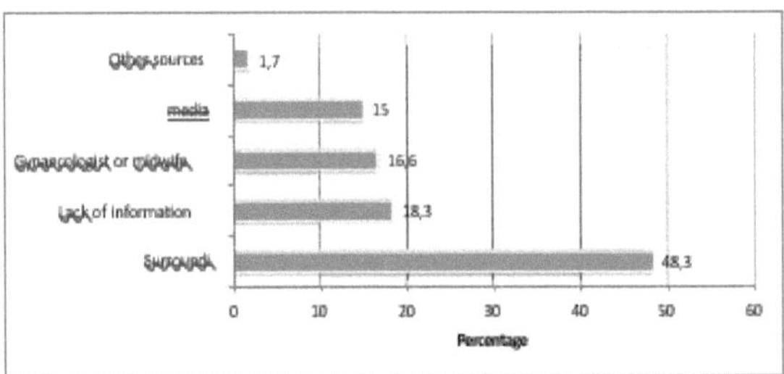

Figure 9: Distribution of parturients according to sources of information about childbirth.

3.5.Complications of pregnancy :

Almost half of all pregnancies (55%) were completed without complications (Figure 10).

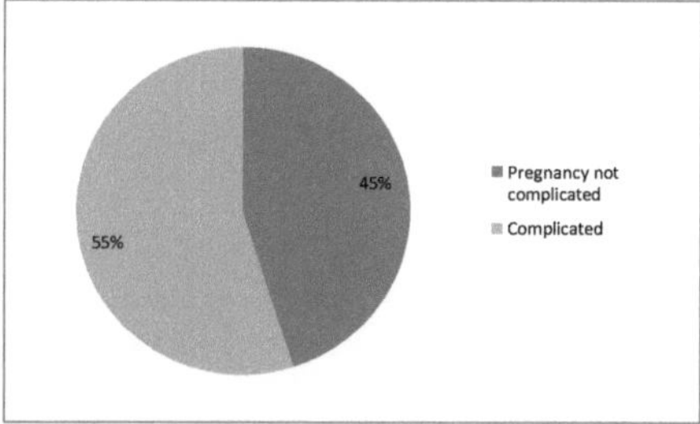

Figure 10: Distribution of parturients according to the presence of dysgravidia.

3.6. Hospitalization during current pregnancy :

In 75% of cases, parturients were not hospitalised during their pregnancy.

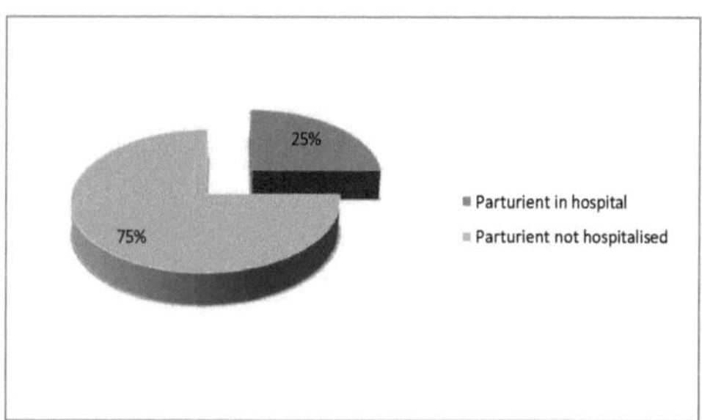

Figure 11: Distribution of parturients according to hospitalisation during current pregnancy.

4. Experience of childbirth :

4.1. Triggering work :

Labour was spontaneous in 73.3% of cases (Figure 12).

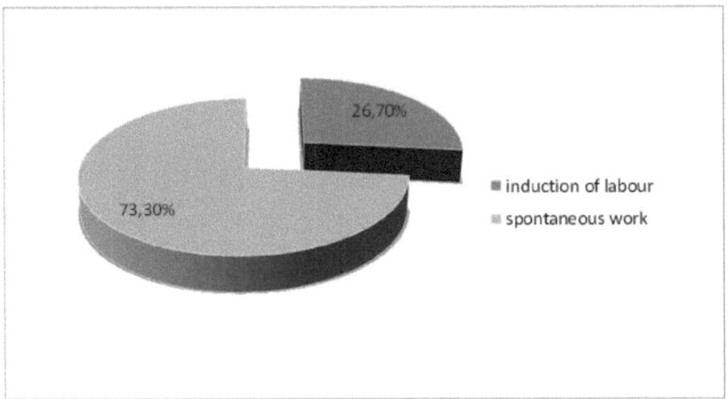

Figure 12: Distribution of parturients according to induction of labour.

4.2. Working hours :

Labour was long in 58.3% of cases (Figure 13).

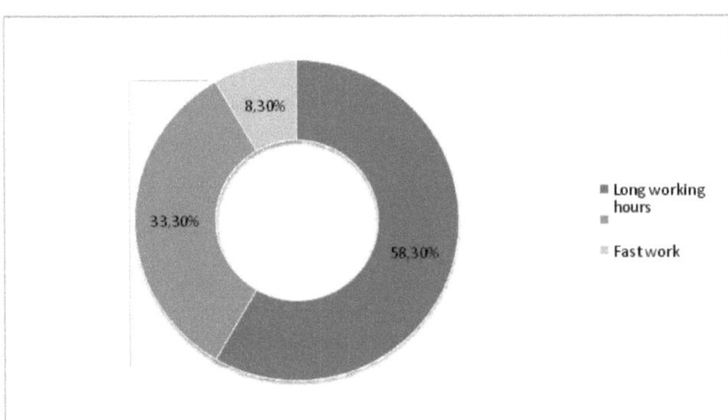

Figure 13: Distribution of parturients according to length of labour.

4.3. Delivery method :

Delivery was instrumental in 56.7% of cases, and emergency caesarean sections accounted for 38.3% of the series (Figure 14).

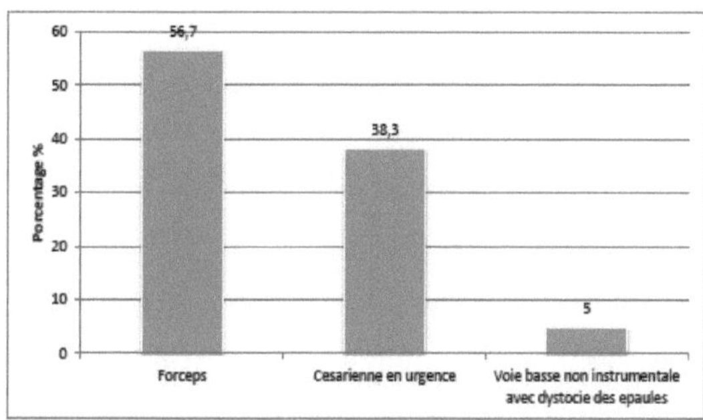

Figure 14: Breakdown of women by mode of delivery.

4.4. Obstetrical indications :

Forceps delivery was indicated for maternal fatigue or insufficient expulsive effort in 41.2% of cases. In addition, 65.2% of caesarean sections were indicated for failure to engage (Table II).

Table II: Distribution of parturients according to the indication for caesarean section or forceps.

Mode delivery	Indication	Number of employees (n)	Percentage (%)
Forceps (n= 34)	Fatigue maternal / expulsive expulsive efforts insufficient	14	41,2
	No increase in presentation	12	35,3
	Acute foetal distress expulsion	8	23,5
Caesarean section emergency (n=23)	Lack of commitment	15	65,2
	Stagnation of the dilatation	6	26
	Acute foetal distress	2	8,7

4.5. Information about the procedure / obstetrical decision :

In 45% of cases, the parturients had judged that they were non sufficiently informed of the procedure performed or the decision taken (Figure 15).

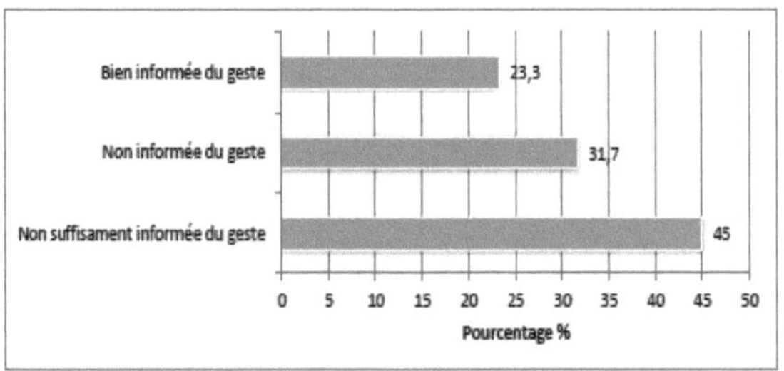

Figure 15: Parturients' assessment of information about the obstetrical procedure or the decision taken.

4.6. Parturient's reaction to the procedure :

The emotion most frequently expressed (55%) was anxiety about the procedure being performed. (Figure 16).

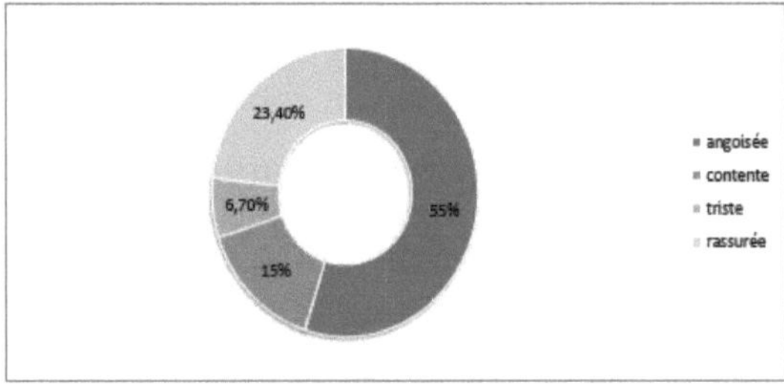

Figure 16: Distribution of parturients according to their reaction to the procedure performed.

4.7. Anaesthesia :

Rachid anaesthesia was used in 35% of parturients. No anaesthetic was used in 36.7% of parturients during instrumental extraction or episiotomy (Figure 17).

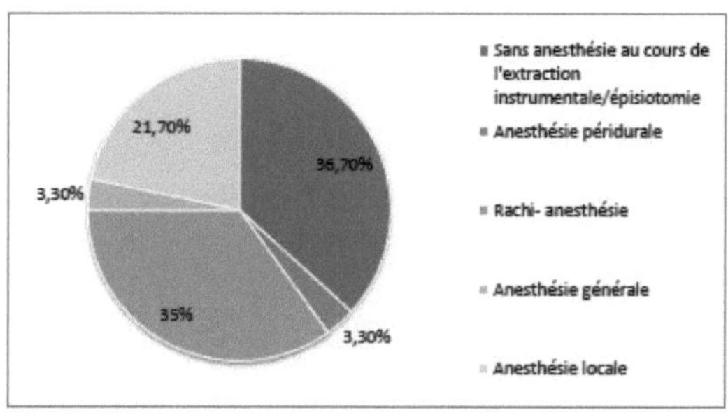

Figure 17: Distribution of parturients according to type of anaesthesia.

4.8. Judgement of parturients concerning violent practices during childbirth :

Verbal abuse was reported by 41.7% of parturients. It seemed that 28.3% of parturients did not feel that they had been subjected to violence during childbirth (Figure 18).

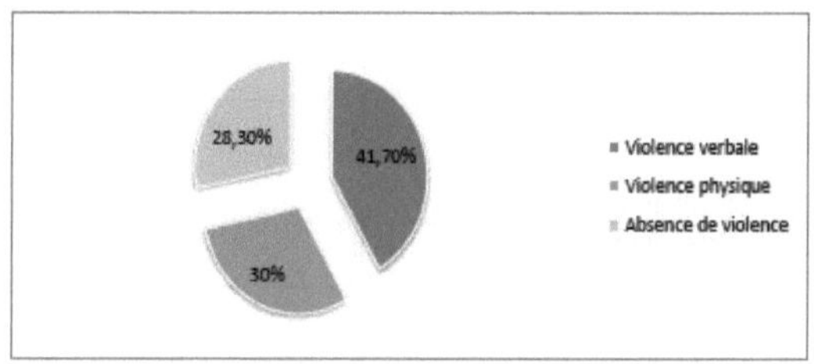

Figure 18: Parturients' assessment of violent practices during childbirth.

4.9.Parturients' opinions of the healthcare team :

Of the parturients questioned, 38.3% felt supported by the healthcare team. Parturients felt that their privacy was not respected in 38.3% of cases and that their pain was not taken into consideration in 43.3% of cases (Figure 19).

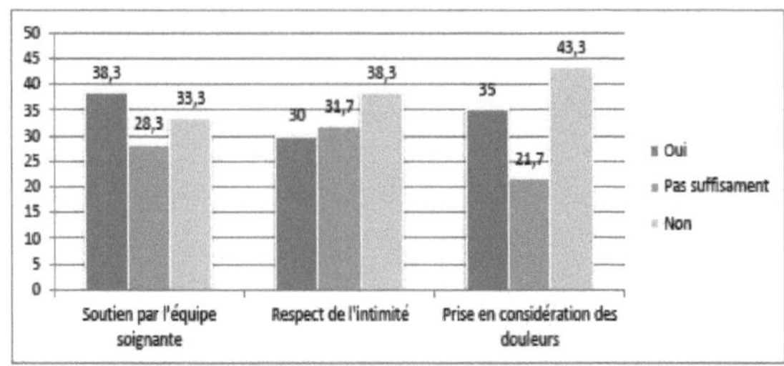

Figure 19: Distribution of parturients according to their opinion of the health care team.

4.10.Complications of childbirth :

Maternal complications were perineal tears in 55.6% of cases. For the newborn, the most frequent complication was neonatal distress (54%) (Table III).

Table III: Distribution of parturients according to delivery complications.

	Complication	Workforce	Percentage
Complication kindergarten (n=18)	Perineal tear	10	55,6
	Uterine inertia	8	44,4
Neonatal complication (n= 26)	Neonatal distress	14	54
	Eye damage	5	19,2
	Facial paralysis	3	11,5
	Subdural haematoma	3	11,5
	Neonatal death	1	3,8

4.11. Overall assessment of childbirth experience by parturients :

Parturients' assessment of their childbirth experience by means of a score rated from 0 to 10 is reported in Table IV.

Table IV: Parturients' assessment of their experience of childbirth.

	Median	Spread- type	extremes
Delivery notes	5	2,9	[0 - 10]
Evaluation of the sensation of fear during childbirth	10	2,3	[0 - 10]
Assessing the quality of care	6 ,5	2,9	[0 - 10]

5. Psychological impact of childbirth :

5.1. Immediate post-partum :

The feeling most expressed by women (38.4%) was recognition (Figure 20).

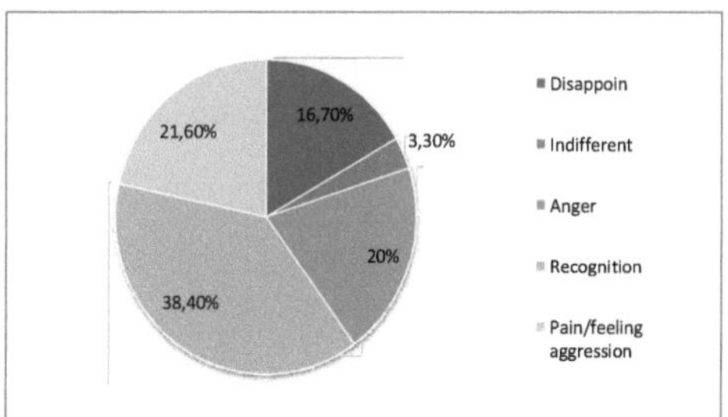

Figure 20: Distribution of women according to feelings in the immediate post-partum period.

5.2.Mother-baby relationship :

The majority of women (81.7%) had breastfed their babies. Furthermore, in terms of judging the mother-baby relationship, the majority of women (80%) reported an appreciation of their baby (Figure 19).

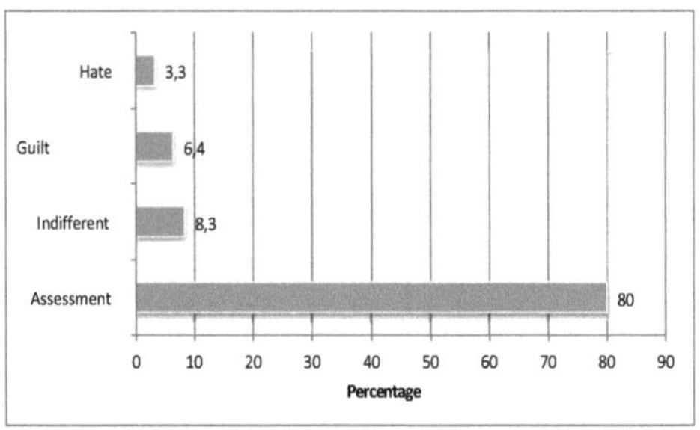

Figure 21: Distribution of women according to their opinion of their relationship with their baby.

5.3. Marital relationship :

After giving birth, 45% of women noted an improvement in their marital relationship (Figure 20).

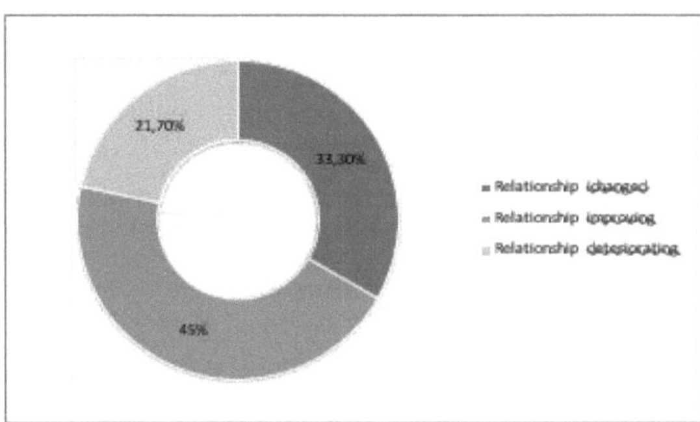

Figure 22: Breakdown of women by changes in their marital relationship.

5.4.Family relationship :

After giving birth, 43.3% of women had unchanged relationships with their loved ones (Figure 23).

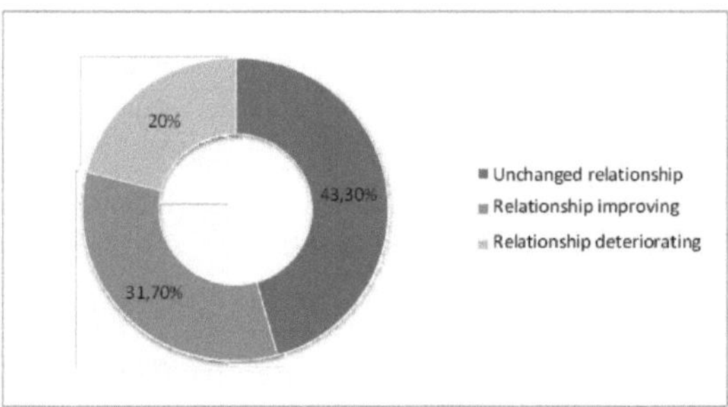

Figure 23: Breakdown of women according to their relationship with their nearest and dearest.

5.5. Women's sex lives :

In 38.3% of cases, women reported a sex life similar to that prior to childbirth. (Figure 24).

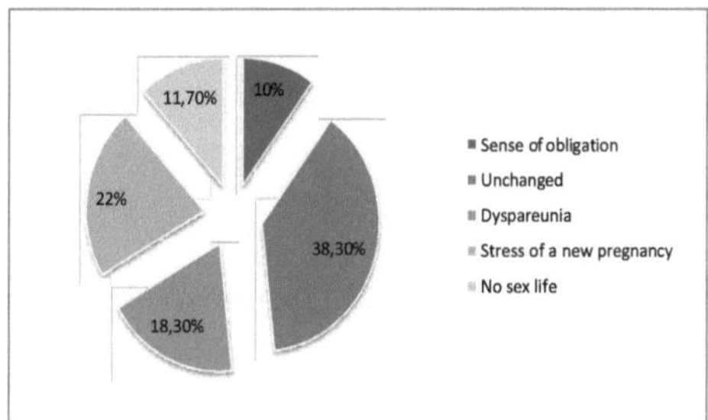

Figure 24: Distribution of women according to changes in their post-partum sex life.

5.6.Post-traumatic stress disorder score according to the IES-R scale :

The mean PTSD score was 29.8 with a standard deviation of 14.8 [4-65]. A score greater than 33, indicating post-traumatic stress disorder, was noted in 41.7% of the women, 35% of whom had a score greater than or equal to 37, indicating severe PTSD (Figure 25).

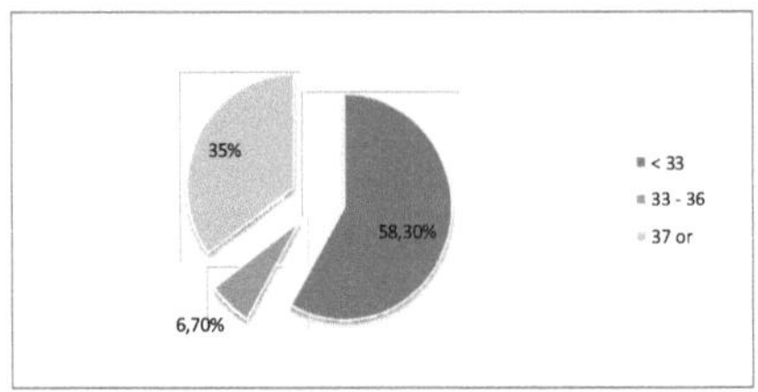

Figure 25: Breakdown of women by PTSD score.

5.7. Depression score according to the Edinburgh Postpartum Depression Scale :

The mean depression score was 11.8 with a standard deviation of 7.3 [2 - 30]. A score greater than or equal to 13, indicating postpartum depression, was noted in 46.7% of women (Figure 26).

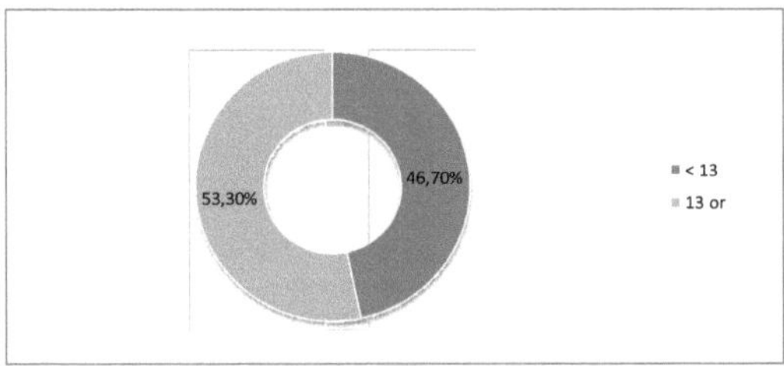

Figure 26: Distribution of women according to post-partum depression score.

5.8. Psychological support :

In 55% of cases, women sought help from family and friends (Figure 27).

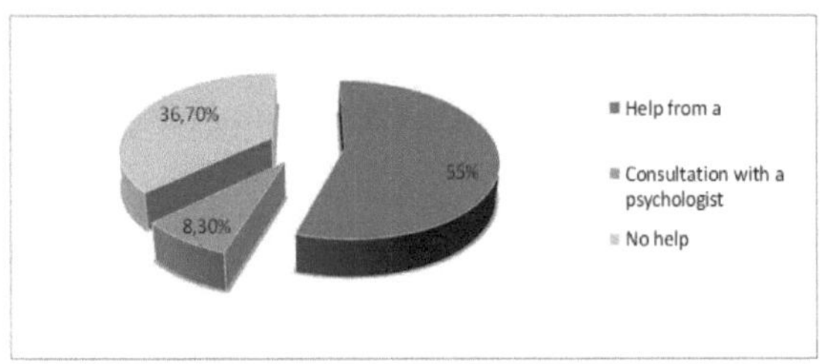

Figure 27: Breakdown of women by request for help.

For the women who had sought help, 48.3% reported an improvement, 11.7% were indifferent and the remaining women (3.3%) reported a worsening of their condition.

5.9.Cause of dystocia according to the woman :

Women thought that experienced dystocia was a physiological phenomenon delivery in 38.3% of cases (Figure 28).

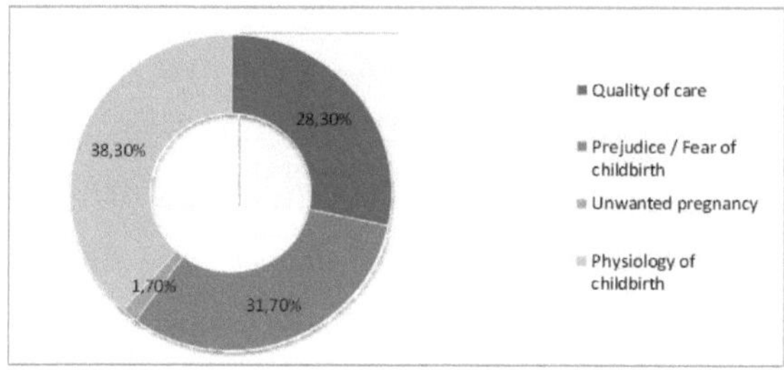

Figure 28: Distribution of women according to their opinion of the cause of dystocia experienced.

5.10. Desire for a new pregnancy :

Almost half of the women (51.7%) expressed a desire to become pregnant again. However, 48.3% did not. As for the attitude to be changed for a subsequent pregnancy, 25% of women wanted to have a birth preparation (Figure 27).

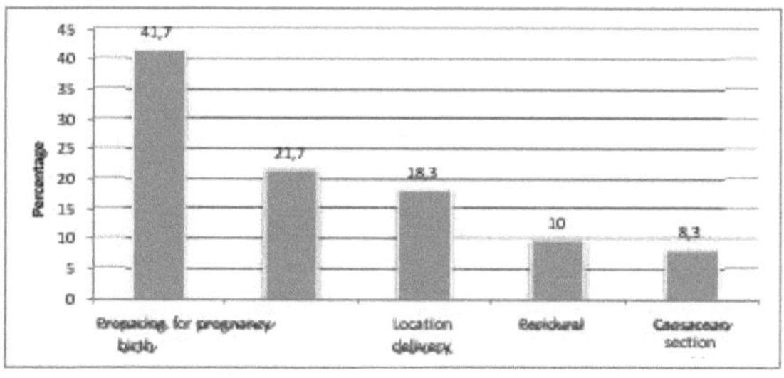

Figure 29: Distribution of women according to the attitude to change for a subsequent pregnancy.

II. Analytical study

1. Uni- analysis

1.1.Factors associated with post-traumatic stress in the case of of obstructed labour:

The PTSD score was higher in primiparous women, with a significant difference (OR=1.5 (0.4 - 2.3), p=0.03). Furthermore, the score was significantly higher if the patient felt unsupported by the nursing team (OR = 3.7 (1.2 - 10.6), p=0.016). The absence of information about the obstetrical procedure significantly increased the risk of PTSD (OR=1.2 (0.4 - 3.5), p=0.04), as did physical or verbal violence during childbirth (OR=1.8 (0.8 - 4), p=0.04). The occurrence of maternal complications after delivery also significantly increased the risk of PTSD (OR=1.7 (1-3), p=0.04). Table V reports the results of the uni-variate analysis of factors associated with PTSD.

Table V: Post-traumatic stress disorder according to women's characteristics, pregnancy and experience of childbirth.

Factor	OR (95% confidence interval) confidence interval (CI))	p
Age (=<30 years versus >30 years)	1,4 (0,5 - 4)	0,33
Origin (urban versus rural)	1,2 (0,4 - 1,7)	0,48
Parity (primiparous versus parity >= 2)	1,5 (0,4 - 2,3)	0,03
Complications of pregnancy (yes versus no)	1,1 (0,4 - 3,1)	0,52
Triggering (yes versus no)	1,1 (0.3 - 3,7)	0,5
Working hours (normal versus abnormal)	0,9 (0,3 - 2,7)	0,53
Mode of delivery (caesarean section vs. caesarean section) instrumental extraction)	3,3 (1 - 10)	0,04
Information about the procedure performed (yes versus no)	1,2 (0,4 - 3,5)	0,04
Violence (yes versus no)	1,8 (0,8 - 4)	0,04
Team support (yes versus no)	3,7(1,2 - 10,6)	0,016
Respect for privacy (yes versus no)	2 (0,7 - 5,8)	0.13
Pain considered (yes versus no)	2,8 (0,97 - 8,2)	0,05
Maternal complication (yes versus no)	1,7 (1 - 3)	0,04
Neonatal complication (yes versus no)	0,5 (0,18 - 1,46)	0,16

1.2.Factors associated with postpartum depression (PPD) in the case of obstructed labour:

The PPD score was significantly higher if the patient felt that she was not supported by the health care team throughout labour and delivery (OR= 5 (1.64 - 15.25), p=0.004) or that her pain was not taken into consideration (OR= 3.9 (1.28 - 11.64), p= 0.014).In addition, the score was significantly higher in the case of emergency caesarean section than in the case of instrumental extraction (OR=2.2 (1 - 4.7), p=0.014) and physical or verbal violence during childbirth significantly increased the risk of PPD (OR=2.04 (0.48 - 8.6), p=0.03). Table VI reports the results of the uni-variate analysis of factors associated with PPD.

Table VI: Post-partum depression according to women's characteristics, pregnancy and experience of childbirth.

Factor	OR (95% CI)	p
Age (:S30 years versus >30 years)	1,1 (0,3 - 3,06)	0,53
Origin (urban versus rural)	1,2 (0,4 - 3,7)	0,5
Parity (primiparous versus parity 2)	0,7 (0,2 - 2,2)	0,4
Complication of pregnancy (yes versus no)	0,85 (0,3 - 0,4)	0,48
Triggering (yes versus no)	1,1 (0,37 - 3,7)	0,5
Working hours (normal versus abnormal)	0,9 (0,3 - 2,7)	0,53
Mode of delivery (caesarean section vs. caesarean section) instrumental extraction)	2,2 (1 - 4,7)	0,014
Information about the procedure performed (yes versus no)	2,2 (0,7 - 6,5)	0,11
Violence (yes versus no)	2,04 (0,48 - 8 ,6)	0,03
Team support (yes versus no)	5 (1,64 - 15,25)	0,004
Respect for privacy (yes versus no)	2,04 (0,7 - 5,8)	0,137
Pain considered (yes versus no)	3,9 (1,28 - 11,64)	0,014
Maternal complication (yes versus no)	0,21 (0,06 - 0,7)	0,4
Neonatal complication (yes versus no)	0,6 (0,24 - 1,9)	0,32

1.3. Relationship between TPS and PLR :

There was a statistically significant correlation between the occurrence of PTSD and PPD (OR=80.6 (14.9 - 435.4), p<0.001) (table VII).

Table VII: Correlation between SPT and DPP.

	OR (95% confidence interval)	p
Correlation between PLR (score	80,6 (14,9 - 435,4)	<0,001

2. Multi- analysis

2.1. Independent factors associated with PTSD in childbirth dystocic

Multi-variate analysis showed no independent factor associated with PTSD after dystocic delivery (Table VIII).

Table VIII: Multivariate analysis of factors associated with PTSD

Factor	OR (95% CI)	p
Parity (primiparous versus parity 2)	1,6 (0,4 - 7,7)	0,4
Mode of delivery (caesarean section versus extraction) instrumental)	1,3 (0,5 - 1,6)	0,2
Information about the procedure performed (yes versus no)	1,3 (0,04 - 2)	0,3
Violence (yes versus no)	1,6 (0,13 - 2,6)	0,5
Consideration of pain (yes versus no)	1,2 (0,15- 5,4)	0,3
Team support (yes versus no)	2,6 (0,7 - 8,6)	0,1
Maternal complications of childbirth (yes versus no)	1,2 (0,6 - 1,1)	0,3

2.2.Independent factors associated with PPD in childbirth dystocic.

In multivariate analysis, the only independent factor associated with PPD was the patient's judgement not to be supported by the nursing team (p=0.03) (table IX).

Table IX: Multivariate analysis of factors associated with PPD

Factor	OR (95% CI)	p
Mode of delivery (caesarean section versus extraction) instrumental)	0,6 (0,1 - 3,2)	0,5
Violence (yes versus no)	0,7 (0,17 - 3,1)	0,7
Team support (yes versus no)	3,6 (1 - 11)	0,03
Consideration of pain (yes versus no)	2,1 (0,4 -10,6)	0,3

DISCUSSION

I. Epidemiological characteristics and obstetrics

1. Age

In our study, the mean age was 29.1 years [19-40 years]. The most common age groups were 20-29 (46.7%) and 30-39 (47.6%). On the other hand, in the study by Kjaergaard et al, the over-35 age group was the most frequent in cases of dystocic delivery(31) . The study published by Waldenström et al. also showed that age over 40 was more frequent in cases of dystocic delivery(32) .
In the series by Dimassi et al. studying Tunisian women's experience of childbirth, the average age of parturients was 30.4 years(33) . In fact, this is the age of intense sexual activity in our country, and therefore of procreation, and this may explain the discrepancy between our results and those reported in the literature.

2. Parity

Primiparity has been reported as a risk factor for dystocic labour. In the study by Selin et al.(34) , primiparous women accounted for 77.5% of patients with a dystocic delivery, with a significantly higher risk than multiparous women ($p<0.001$). Also, in the series by Sheiner et al, most patients were primiparous and the risk of dystocia increased significantly in the case of primiparity (OR = 3.8, 95% CI 3.3-4.3)(35) . In our study, similarly, primiparous women represented 71.7% of the series.

3. Complications of pregnancy

In our study, 55% of pregnancies were uncomplicated and 75% of women were not hospitalised during pregnancy. On the other hand, Sheiner et al. reported that parturients with pregnancy complications such as arterial hypertension or hydramnios were at greater risk of dystocic labour[35] . A review of the literature also reported that the risk of dystocia increased in pregnancies complicated by foetal anomalies such as macrosomia[36] .

4. Mode of work

Labour was spontaneous in 73.3% of parturients who had a dystocic birth in our series. In this context, Boulvain et al. reported that induction of labour significantly reduced the risk of dystocia ($p=0.004$)[37] . Sanchez et al also demonstrated that induced labour was associated with a lower rate of emergency caesarean sections (20.1% versus 22.0%, OR 0.88; 95% CI 0.78, 0.99)[38] .

II. Experiences of childbirth

In our study, 45% of parturients said they were not informed of the procedure and 55% of parturients reported anxiety about the birth experience. In the immediate post-partum period, 58.3% of women expressed negative feelings such as disappointment, anger and pain. In Dimassi's Tunisian study, 48.5% of women found childbirth to be a traumatic experience, especially the conditions in the delivery room[33] . In contrast, a study by Boorman et al in Australia reported only 19.7% traumatic birth experiences[39] . However, the rate reported by Alcorn et al was 45.5%[40] .

Although some authors, such as Tham et al, have stated that childbirth, whatever its outcome, can be a traumatic experience[41] , consideration of the conditions of childbirth is necessary to ensure that this significant event takes place without negative consequences for the parturient.

III. Post-traumatic stress disorder (PTSD) and post-partum depression (PPD) after dystocic delivery.

During the postpartum period, women are particularly vulnerable to a wide variety of psychological disorders, and this risk may be increased in the event of a difficult delivery. In our study, we assessed the psychological impact of obstructed labour in terms of PTSD and/or PPD.

1. Prevalence

1.1. Post-traumatic stress disorder

Our study found a 41.7% prevalence of post-partum PTSD, and 35% of women had severe PTSD after a dystocic delivery. It has been reported in the literature that PTSD can occur following a traumatic birth(42) . In this context, several studies have assessed the prevalence of PTSD: the most recent was conducted by Montmasson et al. and published in 2020, which found a prevalence of 13.6% of postpartum PTSD, partly explained by the fact that their sample consisted solely of primiparous women(43) .

In addition, the study by Yildiz et al, published in 2017, noted a prevalence of 18.5% in a so-called "high-risk" sample, and a prevalence of 43% at 4 months over a period from immediate postpartum to 14 months after delivery(44) .

The variations in prevalence between the different studies and the rate noted in our series can be explained by the variability of the inclusion criteria between the studies (non-inclusion of women with a history of psychiatric pathology or antenatal depression, inclusion of women who had a dystocic delivery at least 3 months previously).

1.2. Post partum depression

In our study, we found that 53.3% of women had experienced PPD. The occurrence of PPD was significantly correlated with a high PTSD score (p<0.001). According to the study by Stander et al, published in 2014, the two disorders may result from a common vulnerability or common risk factors[45] . Another study, by Contractor et al and published in 2018, explained the comorbidity between PTSD and depression in part by a causal relationship between the two disorders, such that the development of PTSD may lead to depression or vice versa[46] .

In a Tunisian study published in 2014 by Masmoudi et al, the percentage of occurrence of depression after eight weeks of childbirth was 12.6%[47] .

According to the literature, the prevalence of PPD varies from 10 to 20%, with an average prevalence of 13%[48,49] .

These results were not consistent with those reported in our study. In fact, the other studies had a larger and more diversified sample, whereas our study was limited to women who had experienced a dystocic birth, which in the women's opinion was a traumatic event and a major factor associated with post-partum depression.

2. Factors associated with PTSD and PPD after obstructed labour

2.1. Factors linked to the characteristics of the population of study

- **Age**

Our study showed that the average age of parturients was 29.1 years. The analytical study showed no significant difference between age and the occurrence of PTSD or PPD (p=0.33 and p=0.53 respectively). Similarly, a 2014 Tunisian series investigating postpartum depression in 302 women reported that the most common age range was 25-35 years[47] . Another study by Levinson et al. in the United States reported that the risk of postpartum depressive disorders increased with younger maternal age[50] . In addition, another study by Carina et al. showed that the risk of developing PTSD increased with maternal age[51] .

- **Socio-economic characteristics**

In our study, 45% of the women had completed secondary education, 56.7% were housewives and 90% of the parturients were of average socio-economic status. Urban or rural origin had no statistically significant impact on the occurrence of PTSD (p=0.48) or PPD (p=0.5). A Tunisian study by Masmoudi et al.(47) reported that low socio-economic status and low level of education were risk factors for developing postpartum blues. This study also reported that women with a low socio-economic level were more likely to develop post-partum depression. In addition, according to C. Vedeler et al, women with low socio-economic status, less than tertiary education and housewives were more exposed to negative experiences during labour and birth(52) .

- **Gender and parity :**

Primigravida represented 65% of our series and 71.7% of patients were primiparous. In univariate analysis, primiparity was a factor associated with PTSD in cases of dystocic delivery (p=0.03). In multivariate analysis, primiparous women had a higher risk of PTSD, but the difference was not statistically significant (OR=1.6, p=0.4). On the other hand, primiparity did not seem to correlate with the risk of PPD in our study. Our results were consistent with those reported in the literature. Indeed, the studies carried out by Angelini et al, D. Ertan et al and M. Modarres et al suggested that the majority of women developing PTSD after a traumatic birth were primiparous women(51,53,54) .

2.2. Factors linked to childbirth

- **Delivery method :**

In our study, having an emergency caesarean section during labour appeared to be more associated with PTSD and PPD than the use of instrumental extraction at the end of labour in univariate analysis (p=0.04 and p=0.014 respectively). In multivariate analysis, emergency caesarean section was associated with a higher risk of PTSD but the correlation was not statistically significant (OR= 1.3, p= 0.2). According to J. Carter et al. the mode of delivery was significantly correlated with maternal PTSD symptoms[55] . Another study by Ertan et al. conducted in 2021 assessed PTSD related to childbirth using the CBTS (The City Birth Trauma Scale) and showed that women who had an emergency caesarean section had the highest scores. of PTSD, followed by those with vacuum deliveries and forceps[53] .The study by Lei Sun et al. reported that the mode of delivery had a significant impact on the prevalence of postpartum PPD[56] . By comparing the prevalence of emergency caesarean section and vaginal delivery, this study showed that women who had an emergency caesarean section had a higher risk of developing PPD.

- **Information about the procedure**

Almost half of the women (45%) felt that they had not been sufficiently informed about the procedure or the decision taken. In addition, the emotion most frequently expressed (55%) was anxiety about the procedure. This judgement of not being informed of the procedure performed had a significant impact on the occurrence of PTSD (p=0.04) but not on PPD (p= 0.11). However, according to l. Dupré, there was no direct link between not being informed during pregnancy or labour and patients' overall experience of labour and birth[20] . On the other hand, the same study reported that parturients who were anxious at the announcement had a more negative experience, and that patients who were informed during labour about the future possibilities for their delivery felt more confident and had more control over the event. In this context, Carter et al. showed that compassionate care and the inclusion of women in decision-making processes could have an impact on reducing feelings of anxiety and fear of childbirth[55] . Nyberg et al. also showed that a group of women suffering from postnatal PTSD believed that a lack of support and control during childbirth had caused their PTSD[57] .

- **Support from the care team**

Only 38.3% of the women felt supported by their care team. This lack of support from the care team was linked to a higher risk of PTSD (p=0.016) and PPD (p=0.004) in univariate analysis. In multivariate analysis, the absence of support from the care team was an independent factor associated with PPD (p=0.03). The health care team plays an important role during childbirth, not only in providing the necessary care for the woman and her baby, but also in providing support, listening and information.The study by F. Viirman et al. showed that a lack of trust, support and information, and the exclusion of women from their birth plans by not respecting their choice, could be the cause of a negative birth experience, and the latter was one of the main causes of PTSD[(58)] . Van Heumen et al. showed that women who received support felt protected and supported in the face of possible complications, inconveniences or doubts, which reduced the risk of stress during the post-partum period[(59)] .
In addition, the study by Vera A Yakupova et al. showed that women who received good support during childbirth from their partner, midwives and other healthcare staff were more satisfied with their delivery[(60)] . This satisfaction plays a major role in reducing the risk of PPD.

- **Violence during childbirth**

Our results showed that 41.7% of the women reported verbal violence and 30% reported physical violence. This notion of violence during childbirth was significantly correlated with the occurrence of PTSD (p=0.04) and PPD (p=0.03) in univariate analysis, although this correlation was not significant in multivariate analysis. The study by S. Martinez-Vázquez et al.[(61)] showed that women who had experienced verbal obstetric violence were at greater risk of developing PTSD than women who had experienced psycho-affective obstetric violence. Similarly, the study by Sher Goaz Melet et al. reported that obstetric violence (verbal, physical and psycho-affective) could have a profound psychological impact such as acute postpartum stress disorder (ASD), post-traumatic stress disorder (PTSD) and postpartum depression (PPD)[62] .

- **Pain management**

According to our study, 43.3% of women did not receive anaesthesia during labour, instrumental extraction or episiotomy. This negative perception of pain by women was associated with a higher risk of PTSD (OR=2.8, p=0.05) and PPD (OR=3.9, p=0.014).With regard to the correlation between the perception of pain and PPD, similar to our results, the literature reports that pain during childbirth was one of the risk factors for PPD, and that epidural analgesia could reduce this risk[63,64] .Regarding PTSD, our results were consistent with those of Ghanbari- Homayi et al.[65] who demonstrated that the probability of a traumatic birth experience without analgesia was 4.24 times greater than when using analgesia. However, in the study by J, A Kountanis et al.[66] , positive perception of the pain of childbirth was associated with a reduced risk of probable PTSD at 6 weeks postpartum and after 12 months, but there was no significant relationship between perception of pain and PTSD. Indeed, for some women, the pain of childbirth is not necessarily a negative experience leading to trauma. Educating women to manage their pain can positively modify their assessment of the pain ofchildbirth and reduce the rates of post-partum PTSD.

- **Maternal complications after childbirth**

In our study, 20% of women experienced maternal complications after delivery, the most frequent of which were perineal tears and uterine inertia. The occurrence of maternal complications was associated with a higher risk of PTSD (OR= 1.7, p=0.04). Indeed, it has been reported that women with obstetric complications often have a high risk of developing clinical and mental health disorders (anxiety, panic attacks and PTSD)[67] .

3. Correlation between PTSD and depression :

In our study, we found that post-natal depression was positively correlated with post-traumatic stress symptoms ($p<0.001$). In fact, several studies support this correlation. According to Milen L. Radell et al.[68] symptoms of depression were generally associated with PTSD, with a reciprocal relationship between the two disorders. Despite the overlap of symptoms, the two disorders are distinct entities and depend, at least in part, on distinct biological mechanisms. However, both entities are clearly linked to the psychopathology of stress, with a significant overload of intrusiveness, mood and mood changes.

IV. Dystoic childbirth and psychosocial factors .

1. The impact of childbirth on a woman's daily life :

In the immediate postpartum period, the mother finds it difficult to adapt to her new role: disappointment, feelings of failure, anger, pain and sadness may be expressed. In our study, the most frequently expressed feeling in the postpartum period (38.4%) was gratitude.

2. Mother-child relationship :

Our study showed that the majority of women (81.7%) had breastfed their babies. What's more, when it came to judging the mother-baby relationship, the majority of women (80%) reported an appreciation of their baby. The negative experience or trauma of a complicated birth is likely to influence not only the mother, but also the baby. As a result, the relationship with the baby may be affected: the mother may neglect her child, avoid emotional interactions with him, or even feel hatred towards him[69] . This was indeed reported in the study by Garthus-Niegel et al, published in 2017, according to which maternal PTSD had a negative impact on breastfeeding. Mothers suffering from PTSD were less likely to breastfeed[70] . The discrepancy between our results and those in the literature may be explained by the fact that the women were well cared for by their families. Indeed, 55% of our women asked for help from their relatives and almost half of the women (43.3%) maintained a stable relationship with their families.

3. Marital relationship and sex life :

In our study, the marital relationship was improved in 45% of cases. In terms of sex life, we noted that 38.3% of women had a sex life similar to that before giving birth. However, according to the study by Garthus-Niegel et al conducted in 2018, difficulties could be observed with intimacy or relationships[71] . Another study showed that PTSD was associated with avoidance of sexual relations for fear of giving birth again[72] .

Our results could be explained, according to the women, by the support and harmony within the couple. However, 22% of the women in our series were stressed by the fear of another pregnancy.

V. Recommendations and future prospects :

According to the results of our study, we found that it is essential and compulsory for women to be accompanied and prepared for childbirth and unexpected events during childbirth. In fact, the entire population (100%) had not attended any childbirth preparation classes, and 41.7% of women wished to do so during subsequent pregnancies. In addition, we noted a lack of support and information from the midwife, as almost half the parturients (48.3%) received information from those around them. Similarly, in Dimassi's Tunisian series, 79% of women had recourse to the media and social networks, where dramatic accounts of childbirth were reported[33] .

1. The role of preparation for birth and parenthood :

According to the French National Authority for Health (HAS)[73] , preparation for childbirth used to focus on pain management. It is now moving towards providing comprehensive support for the woman and her partner, encouraging their active participation in the birth process.
The aim of these sessions is to :

- create a bond of trust between the midwife and the parturient.

- to guide, prepare and support the couple in becoming parents.

- Providing clear and accurate information tailored to each situation, and advising women of the risks that may arise during and after childbirth, as well as the alternative methods of childbirth available, namely instrumental extractions and caesarean sections.

- discuss the notion of pain during labour and its progress, childbirth, and methods of relief.

According to the 2021 perinatal survey, 80.3% of primiparous women took part in the birth and parenthood preparation sessions (PNP)[74] .

2. The role of the midwife

The midwife plays an essential role before and after childbirth. She listens, advises, supports, explains and informs the pregnant woman and the couple about the progress of the pregnancy, the birth and its aftermath.
The midwife plays this role during antenatal consultations and birth preparation sessions, as well as during childbirth and the maternity stay. She also plays an important role in screening for post-partum anxiety-depressive disorders and identifying women with PTSD.

3. Action projects :

Psychological support for patients with obstructed labour, foetal/maternal pathologies or who have experienced an unexpected accident during childbirth, during the maternity stay by a psychologist who can screen for post-partum depression and anxiety using a validated tool and then refer the woman to appropriate support structures.

- Offer a systematic early prenatal interview to pregnant women, either individually or as a couple. The aim of this interview is to identify medico-psychosocial problems at an early stage and to enable couples to express their expectations and needs regarding the pregnancy, as well as encouraging them to take part in the PNP. It is also important to explain to women the psychological fragility associated with pregnancy and childbirth, which may be exacerbated in the post-natal period.At the end of our study, the main interest would be to enable better screening of patients at risk of psychological problems linked to the birth process, but also to insist on support and guidance for parturients during these sensitive moments.

VI. Strengths and limitations of our study

One of the strengths of our study was its analytical approach, which enabled us to study the factors associated with psychological problems after dystocic childbirth. This could enable us to define at-risk populations to which special attention should be paid. However, our study was limited by the relatively small size of the sample, partly due to the fact that some of the women could not be contacted or did not cooperate.

CONCLUSION

Because of their frequency and repercussions, post-partum clinical and psychological disorders are a major public health issue, as they affect not only the mother's interactions with her newborn, her partner and her family and friends, but also the patients' quality of life.Our work has provided a global view of the relational, emotional and psychological problems of the post-partum period linked to laborious, dystocic deliveries. This study highlights the importance of the parturient's subjective experience of childbirth and the perception of complications, which are strong predictors of PPD and postpartum PTSD.Subjective experiences of childbirth, obstetric history and stress levels during childbirth are all factors that favour the emergence of postpartum PTSD. Screening for these factors at an early stage enables us to identify the women most at risk of post-partum PTSD and PTSD, so that we can offer them specialised treatment.

APPENDICES

Annex 1: impact of event scale-revised

دائما 4	غالبا 3	احيانا 2	نادرا 1	ابدا 0	
					هل تذكر الحادثة يجعلك تستعيد المشاعر التي احسستها في تلك اللحظة.
					هل لديك مشاكل في البقاء نائما
					هل الاشياء الاخرى تجعلك تفكر في الحادثة.
					هل شعرت بالغضب و سرعة الانفعال.
					لقد تجنبت الانزعاج عندما فكرت في الأمر أو تذكرت به.
					فكرت في الامر عندما لم أقصد ذلك.
					شعرت أنه لم يحدث أو لم يكن حقيقيًا.
					تجنبت الاشياء التي تفكرني بذلك.
					وجود صور و ذكريات الحادثة في مخيلتي.
					كنت متوتره وخائفة دون سبب وجيه.
					حاولت عدم التفكير في الامر.
					كنت أعلم أنه لا يزال لدي الكثير من المشاعر حيال ذلك ، لكنني لم اواجههم.
					مشاعري حول الحادث كانت شبه مجمده.
					شعرت وأنني اتصرف كما لو كنت لا ازال في الحادثة.
					كان لدي مشكلة في النوم.
					شعرت بموجات من مشاعر شديده عن الحادثة.
					حاولت محو ذلك من ذاكرتي.
					اجد مشاكل في التركيز.
					تذكر الحادثة يتسبب لي في ردود فعل جسدية مثل التعرق صعوبة في التنفس او الغثيان.
					كنت احلم بالحادثة.
					لقد شعرت انني مراقب و على استعداد.
					لقد تجنبت الحديث عن الحادثة.

Appendix 2: Edinburgh depression scale

1. لقد كنت قادرة على الضحك و رؤية الجانب المشرق من الأشياء
بالمقدار نفسه الذي استطعته من قبل
ليس تماما بالمقدار نفسه
قطعا ليس بالمقدار نفسه
كلا، مطلقا

2. لقد تطلعت إلى الأمور بتمتع.
بالمقدار نفسه مثل أي وقت مضى
أقل نوعا ما مما إعتدته
أقل قطعا مما إعتدته
ابدا

3. لقد لمت نفسك دون داع عندما سارت الأمور على غير ما يرام
نعم في معظم الأحيان
نعم في بعض الأحيان
ليس في أحوال كثيرة
كلا، أبدا

4. لقد كنت قلقة و مشغولة البال دون سبب وجيه
كلا،أبدا
نادرا
نعم في بعض الأحيان
نعم في أحوال كثيرة

5. قد شعرت بالخوف و الذعر دون سبب وجيه
نعم، أكثر الأحيان
نعم، في بعض الأحيان
كلا، ليس كثيرا
كلا،أبدا

6. تراكمت الأعمال عليّ، فلم أستطع القيام بها كلها
نعم، في معظم الأحيان
نعم، في بعض الأحيان لم أستطع القيام بها كالمعتاد
كلا، لقد إستطعت القيام بها في بعض الأحيان
كلا، لقد استطعت القيام بها كالمعتاد

7. شعرت بالحزن الشديد لدرجة أنني واجهت صعوبة في النوم
نعم، في معظم الأحيان
نعم، في بعض الأحيان
ليس كثيرا
كلا، أبدا

8. لقد شعرت أنني حزينة أو بائسة
نعم، في معظم الأحيان
نعم في بعض الأحيان
كلا، ليس أكثر الأحيان
كلا، أبدا

9. قد كنت غير سعيدة و شعرت بألم مرير لدرجة أنني كنت أبكي
نعم، في معظم الأحيان
نعم، أكثر الأحيان
فقط من وقت إلى آخر
كلا، أبدا

10. لقد خطرت لي فكره إلحاق الأذى بنفسي
نعم، أكثر الأحيان
نعم، في بعض الأحيان
نادرًا
كلا، مطلقا

REFERENCES

1: Akta S, Ayd n R. The analysis of negative birth experiences of mothers: a qualitative study. J Reprod Infant Psychol. 2019;37(2):176-92.

2: Darvill R, Skirton H, Farrand P. Psychological factors that impact on women's experiences of first-time motherhood: A qualitative study of the transition. Midwifery. 2010;26(3):357-66.

3 :Ayers S. Delivery as traumatic event: prevalence, risk factors, and treatment for postnatal posttraumatic stress disorder. Clin Obstet Gynecol. 2004; 47 (3): 552-67.

4: Molgora S, Fenaroli V, Saita E. The association between childbirth experience and mother's parenting stress: The mediating role of anxiety and depressive symptoms. Women Heal. 2020;60(3):341-51.

5: Bell AF, Andersson E. The birth experience and women's postnatal depression: A systematic review. Midwifery. 2016;39:112-23.

6: Dekel S, Stuebe C, Dishy G. Childbirth induced posttraumatic stress syndrome: A systematic review of prevalence and risk factors. Front Psychol. 2017;8(APR):1-10

6: Chabbert M, Wendland J. The experience of childbirth and perceived sense of control by women during delivery: impact on early mother-infant. Rev médecine périnatale. 2016;8(4):199-206

7: Garthus-Niegel S, Horsch A, Handtke E, von Soest T, Ayers S, Weidner K, et al. The impact of postpartum posttraumatic stress and depression symptoms on couples' relationship satisfaction: A population-based prospective study. Front Psychol. 2018;9(SEP):1-10.

8: World Health Organization. Care in normal birth. Geneva: WHO; 1996. http://apps.who.int/iris/bitstream/10665/63167/1/WHO _FRH_MSM_96.24.pdf.

9: HAS, Normal childbirth: physiological support and medical interventions,

2018.

10: J.-P. Schaal, D. Riethmuller, Dystocies osseuses, 2009.

11: D. Riethmuller, N. Mottet, P.-L. Forey, V. Equy, P. Hoffmann, Dystocies of the soft tissues, 2021.

12: D. Riethmuller, Dynamic dystocia, 2012

13: Julie S. Moldenhauer, MD, Fetal Dystocia, 2021

14: The RPNA team, LES EXTRACTIONS INSTRUMENTALES, 2021.

15: Text of recommendations for clinical practice. Journal of Obstetrics, Gynaecology and Reproductive Biology, 2008; 37: S297-S300.

16: Beucher, G. Maternal complications of instrumental extractions. Journal de Gynécologie Obstétrique et Biologie de la reproduction, 2008; 37: 244-259.

17: Baud O. Neonatal complications of instrumental extractions. Journal de Gynécologie Obstétrique et Biologie de la Reproduction, 2008; 37: 260-268.

18: Pierre F, Rudigoz R-C. Emergency caesarean section: is there an ideal delay? Journal de Gynécologie Obstétrique et Biologie de la Reproduction, 2008; 37, 41-47.

19: HAS, Caesarean section, 2013.

20: Laura DUPRE, INFORMATIONS ET SATISFACTIONS DE L'ACCOUCHEMENT DYSTOCIQUE, 2012.

21: S. Bydlowski. Postpartum psychological disorders: screening and prevention after birth: recommendations. J Gynécologie Obstétrique Biol Reprod. 31 Oct 2015;(44):1152-6. A.M. Bergant et al.
Early postnatal depressive mood: associations with obstetric and psychosocial factors

22: CNGOF, Chapter 35 Item 67 - UE 3 - Pregnancy and post partum psychological disorders, 2016.

23: Pregnancy and post-partum psychological disorders, Child Psychiatry

Department, CHU Angers.
24: Isserlis C., Sutter-Dallay A.L., Dugnat M., Glangeaud-Freudenthal N. Guide pour la pratique de l'entretien prénatal précoce et l'accompagnement psychique des femmes devenus mères. Toulouse, Erès, 2008: 89-128 p.
25: Rozic P.R., Schvartzman J.A. et al. Screening for symptoms of depression during postpartum and the long term follow up: temporal stability and associated factors. Vertex, 2012; 23(106): 409-17e depression
26: American Psychiatric Association (ed). Diagnostic and Statistical Manual of Mental Disorders. Washington, DC: American Psychiatric Press; 1994.
27: J L Cox, J M Holden, R Sagovsky, Detection of postnatal depression. Development of the 10-item Edinburgh Postnatal Depression Scale, 1987.
28: Validation of the Arabic version of the Edinburgh Postnatal Depression Scale and prevalence of postnatal depression on an Algerian sample. Revue EL-Bahith en Sciences Humaines et Sociales, Volume 12 (01) 2020, Algérie : Université Kasdi Marbah Ouargla, (P.P 349-358)
29: Weiss, D.S., & Marmar, C.R. (1997). The Impact of Event Scale-Revised. In J.P. Wilson & T.M. Keane (Eds.), Assessing Psychological Trauma and PTSD (pp.399-411). New York: Guilford.

30: Grazia Ceschi, Arnaud Pictet, Appendix 3. Event impact scale, version (Impact of Event Scale - revised; IES-R-F), 2018.

31: Kjaergaard H, Olsen J, Ottesen B, Dykes AK. Incidence and outcomes of dystocia in the active phase of labor in term nulliparous women with spontaneous labor onset. Acta Obstet Gynecol Scand. 2009;88(4):402-7.
32: Waldenström U, Ekéus C. Risk of labor dystocia increases with maternal age irrespective of parity: a population-based register study. Acta Obstet Gynecol Scand. 2017 Sep;96(9):1063-1069.
33: Kaouther Dimassi , Farah Benzina , Amal Ksouri, Ben Zina Emna , Najla Kamassi , Amira Rakkam , Hejer Selmi , Souad Trabelsi , Amel Triki, Rim

Rafraf . Pregnancy and childbirth: what do Tunisian women experience? MEDICAL TUNISIA - 2020
Vol 98 (n°07).

34: Selin L, Wallin G, Berg M. Dystocia in labour - risk factors, management and outcome: a retrospective observational study in a Swedish setting. Acta Obstet Gynecol Scand. 2008;87(2):216-21.
35: Sheiner E, Levy A, Feinstein U, Hallak M, Mazor M. Risk factors and outcome of failure to progress during the first stage of labor: a population-based study. Acta Obstet Gynecol Scand. 2002 Mar.
36: Lowe NK. A review of factors associated with dystocia and cesarean section in nulliparous women. J Midwifery Womens Health. 2007 May-Jun;52(3):216-28.
37: Boulvain M, Senat MV, Perrotin F, Winer N, Beucher G, Subtil D, Bretelle F, Azria E, Hejaiej D, Vendittelli F, Capelle M, Langer B, Matis R, Connan L, Gillard P, Kirkpatrick C, Ceysens G, Faron G, Irion O, Rozenberg P; Groupe de Recherche en Obstétrique et Gynécologie (GROG). Induction of labour versus expectant management for large-for-date fetuses: a randomised controlled trial. Lancet. 2015 Jun.
38: Sanchez-Ramos L, Olivier F, Delke I, Kaunitz AM. Labor induction versus expectant management for postterm pregnancies: a systematic review with meta-analysis. Obstet Gynecol. 2003.
39: Boorman RJ, Devilly GJ, Gamble J, Creedy DK, Fenwick J. Childbirth and criteria for traumatic events. Midwifery. 2014 Feb;30(2):255-61.
40: Alcorn, K.L., O'Donovan, A., Patrick, J.C., Devilly, G.J., 2010. A prospective longitudinal study of the prevalence of post-traumatic stress disorder resulting from childbirth events. Pyschological Medicine 40, 1849-1859.

41: Tham V, Ryding EL, Christensson K. Experience of support among mothers with and without post-traumatic stress symptoms following emergency

caesarean section. Sex Reprod Healthc. 2010 Nov;1(4):175-80.
42: Stramrood CAI, Huis in 'T Veld EMJ, Van Pampus MG, Berger LWAR, Vingerhoets AJJM, Schultz WCMW, et al. Measuring posttraumatic stress following childbirth: a critical evaluation of instruments. J Psychosom Obstet Gynecol. 2010;31(1):40-9.
43: H Montassmon et al. Factors associated with posttraumatic stress disorder in primiparous women. 2020.
44: Yildiz PD, Ayers S, Phillips L. The prevalence of posttraumatic stress disorder in pregnancy and after birth: A systematic review and meta-analysis. J Affect Disord. 2017;208:634-45.
45: Stander, V.A., Thomsen, C.J., and Highfill-McRoy, R.M. (2014). Etiology of depression comorbidity in combat-related PTSD: a review ofthe literature. Clin. Psychol. Rev. 34: 87- 98.
46: Contractor, A.A., Greene, T., Dolan, M., and Elhai, J.D. (2018). Relationships between PTSD and depression symptom clusters in samples differentiated by PTSD diagnostic status. J. Anxiety.
47: J masmoudi et al. la dépression du postpartum : prévalence et facteurs de risque etude prospective concernant 302 parturientes tunisiennes.2014.
48: Ayers S, Wright DB, Thornton A. Development of a Measure of Postpartum PTSD: The City Birth Trauma Scale. Front Psychiatry. 2018;9:409.
49: Grekin R, O'Hara MW. Prevalence and risk factors of postpartum posttraumatic stress disorder: A meta-analysis. Clin Psychol Rev. 2014;34(5):389-401.
50: Michelle Levinson, Boriana Parvez, David Aboudi, Shetal Shah, Impact of maternal stressors and neonatal clinical factors on postpartum depression screening scores, J Matern Fetal Neonatal Med (2020).
51: Carina R. Angelini, C. Pacagnella, Mary, A. Parpinelli, Carla Silveira, Carla B. Andreucci, Elton C. Ferreira, Juliana P. Santos, Dulce M. Zanardi, Renato T. Souza, Jose G. Cecatti, Post-Traumatic Stress Disorder and severe maternal

morbidity: is there an association?", Clinics (Sao Paulo). 2018; 73: e309.
52: Carina Vedeler, Tine Schauer Eri, Roy Miodini Nilsen, Ellen Blix, Soo Downe, Kjetil A van der Wel, Anne Britt Vika Nilsen, Women's negative childbirth experiences and socioeconomic factors: Results from the Babies Born better survey, (2023).

53: Deniz Ertan, Coraline Hingray, Elena Burlacu, Aude Sterlé and Wissm El-Hage, Post- traumatic stress disorder following childbirth, (2021).
54: Maryam Modarres, Sedigheh Afrasiabi, Parvin Rahnama, Ali Montazeri, Prevalence and risk factors of childbirth-related post-traumatic stress symptoms (2012).
55: Jemima Carter, Debra Bick, Daniel Gallacher, Yan-Shing Chang, Mode of birth and development of maternal postnatal post-traumatic stress disorder: A mixed-methods systematic review and meta-analysis, (2022).
56: Lei Sun, Su Wang, Xi-Qian Li, Association between mode of delivery and postpartum depression: A systematic review and network meta-analysis, (2021).
57: Nyberg, K., Lindberg, I., & Öhrling, K. (2010). Midwives' experience of encountering women with posttraumatic stress symptoms after childbirth. Sexual & Reproductive Healthcare: Official Journal Of The Swedish Association Of Midwives, 1(2), 55-60.
58: Frida Viirman, Andrea Hess Engstrom, Josefin Sjomark, Susanne Hesselman,Inger Sundstrom Poromaa, Lisa Ljungman, Agneta Skoog Svanberg, Anna Wikman, Negative childbirth experience in relation to mode of birth and events during labour: A mixed methods study, European Journal of Obstetrics and Gynecology 282 (2023) 146-154.
59: Mark A. van Heumen, Martine H. Hollander, Maria G. van Pampus, Jeroen van Dillen, and Claire A. I. Stramrood3, Psychosocial Predictors of Postpartum Posttraumatic Stress Disorder in Women With a Traumatic Childbirth Experience, Front Psychiatry. 2018; 9: 348. 60: Vera A Yakupova, Anna Suarez, Postpartum Depression and Birth Experience in Russia, (2021).

61: Sergio Martinez-Vázquez, Julián Rodríguez-Almagro, Antonio Hernández-Martínez, and Juan Miguel Martínez-Galiano, Factors Associated with Postpartum Post-Traumatic Stress Disorder (PTSD) Following Obstetric Violence: A Cross-Sectional Study, J Pers Med. 2021 May; 11(5): 338.
62: Sher Goaz Melet, Noa Feldman, Anna Padoa, [OBSTETRIC VIOLENCE - SINCE WHEN AND WHERE TO: IMPLICATIONS AND PREVENTIVE STRATEGIES] (2022).
63: Daniele C Parise, Caitlin Gilman, Matthew A Petrilli, Dolores Malaspina, Childbirth Pain and Post-Partum Depression: Does Labor Epidural Analgesia Decrease This Risk? (2021).
64: Jianlan Mo, Zhipeng Ning, Xiaoxia Wang, Feng Lv , Jifeng Feng, Linghui Pan, Association between perinatal pain and postpartum depression: A systematic review and meta-analysis (2022).

65: Solmaz Ghanbari-Homayi, Zahra Fardiazar, Shahla Meedya, Sakineh Mohammad- Alizadeh-Charandabi, Mohammad Asghari-Jafarabadi, Eesa Mohammadi and Mojgan Mirghafourvand, Predictors of traumatic birth experience among a group of Iranian primipara women: a cross sectional study, Ghanbari-Homayi et al. BMC Pregnancy and Childbirth (2019) 19:182.
66: Joanna A Kountanis, Robyn Kirk, Jonathan E Handelzalts, Jennifer M Jester, Ros Kirk, Maria Muzik, The associations of subjective appraisal of birth pain and provider-patient communication with postpartum-onset PTSD, Arch Womens Ment Health. 2022 Feb;25(1):171-180.
67: Lisa Hinton, Louise Locock, Marian Knight, Support for mothers and their families after life-threatening illness in pregnancy and childbirth: a qualitative study in primary care, Br J Gen Pract. 2015 Sep;65(638):e563-9.
68: Milen L. Radell, Eid Abo Hamza and Ahmed A. Moustafa, Depression in post-traumatic stress disorder, (2020).
69: Wijma K. Why focus on "fear of childbirth"? J Psychosom Obstet Gynaecol 2003; 24(3):141-3.

70: Ayers S, Eagle A, Waring H. The effects of childbirth-related post-traumatic stress disorder on women and their relation-ships: a qualitative study. Psychol Health Med 2006; 11(4): 389-98.
71: Garthus-Niegel S, Horsch A, Ayers S, Junge-Hoffmeister J, Weidner K, Eberhard-Gran M.(2017). The influence of postpartum PTSD on breastfeeding: A longitudinal population- based study. Birth, 00,1-9. DOI: 10.1111/birt.12328.
72: Garthus-Niegel S, Horsch A, Handtke E, von Soest T, Ayers S, Weidner K, et al. (2018).The Impact of Postpartum Posttraumatic Stress and Depression Symptoms on Couples'Relationship Satisfaction: A Population-Based Prospective Study. Front Psychol, 9, 1-10.DOI: 10.3389/fpsyg.2018.01728.
73: HAS, Preparation for birth and parenthood (PNP), PROFESSIONAL RECOMMENDATIONS, November
74: NATIONAL PERINATAL SURVEY, BIRTHS, FOLLOW-UP AT TWO MONTHS AND THREE MONTHS ESTABLISHMENTS Situation and trends since 2016, October 2022.

SUMMARY

Introduction: *Postpartum psychological disorders are common and may be exacerbated after obstructed labour. Our objectives were to evaluate the factors associated with post-traumatic stress disorder (PTSD), post-partum depression (PPD) and relational aspects after a dystocic delivery.*

Materials and methods: *A descriptive and analytical cross-sectional study including 60 women with dystocic childbirth from July to December 2022 at the Hedi Chaker University Hospital in Sfax.*

Results: *PTSD and PPD were noted in 41.7% and 46.7% of cases. The factors associated with these disorders were primiparity (p=0.03), urgent caesarean section (p=0.04), lack of support (p= 0.016), lack of information (p=0.04), obstetric violence (p=0.04), lack of analgesia (0.05) and maternal complications (p=0.04). Sexual problems were reported in 61.7% of cases and the mother-baby relationship was satisfactory in 80% of cases.*

Conclusion: *Psychological support for patients at risk of mental disorders after a dystocic childbirth is necessary, as is preparation for the birth of pregnant women.*

Key words*: Dystocic delivery, Post-partum, Depression, Post-traumatic stress disorder*

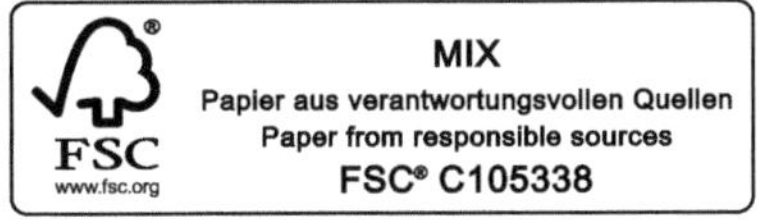

Printed by Books on Demand GmbH, Norderstedt / Germany